The Glucose Solution

A Guide to Transformative Blood Sugar Balance

Jessica Morgan

Table of Contents

Introduction

Emily, a thirty year old worker dealing with the daily rush of tasks, meetings, and the constant buzz of messages on her smartphone, lived in the busy center of a modern city. Emily took joy in her ability to multitask, merging the responsibilities of work and a social life as a driven business woman.

Yet, beyond the surface of her activity and vivacity, a subtle undercurrent of tiredness and unexplainable mood swings interrupted her usually lively existence. Emily, like many others caught up in the hurry and bustle of modern life, had unknowingly gotten removed from a vital component of her health: her blood sugar level.

Emily was sitting at her computer, engaged in a seemingly endless stream of emails, when she was struck by a strange feeling of sleepiness. The sparkling excitement that had driven her morning had faded, leaving her tired and irritated. It was as if her body had found a tripping block in protest.

This was not a one-off event. Emily's journey was filled with occasional energy crashes, each one leaving her confused. A trip to the doctor only added to her confusion: her blood sugar levels were within the "normal" range, but her energy rollercoaster remained a secret.

Emily started on a personal investigation in search of solutions, studying and trying with lifestyle changes, food tweaks, and stress management measures. Slowly, the puzzle parts started to fall into place. Emily began to understand her blood sugar levels' complex dance, learning that they held the key to releasing continuous energy, mental clarity, and emotional well-being.

Emily's situation is not rare. In our fast-paced society, countless individuals are involved in a similar struggle: they look healthy on the surface, but are battling with the underlying fluctuations of blood sugar imbalance. "The Glucose Solution" is the result of numerous Emilys' combined experiences, a guide meant to explain the frequently ignored relationship between our daily actions and the delicate balance of our blood sugar. It's a trip that we can all connect to: one of understanding, balance, and recovering our inner power.

Emily noticed the huge effect of her living choices as she dove more into her studies of blood sugar dynamics. The foods she ate, the amount of stress she carried, and even the quality of her sleep were all finely sewn into the fabric of her health. Emily began to make conscious changes, changing her relationship with food and accepting thoughtful activities that fed her body and soul, equipped with new facts.

The trip was not without its challenges. Breaking free from the ties of easy meals and refusing the draw of stress-induced coffee fixes took patience. Emily, on the other hand, felt a rush of excitement with each tiny success. Her once shifting energy levels had stabilized, and the veil of mental tiredness had lifted. Emily's journey turned into one of strength, showing that with knowledge and effort, one can change the story of their health.

"The Glucose Solution" is a collection of tales like Emily's—stories of finding, change, and victory against our bodies' subtle opponents. It stresses that the difficulties of blood sugar instability are not limited to a small set of individuals, but rather connect with a vast patchwork of people managing the details of modern life.

For those seeking understanding and power over their health journey, this book is a ray of hope. Whether you're dealing with a medical diagnosis, trying to avoid future health issues, or simply wanting a more vibrant life, "The Glucose Solution" gives a helping hand to guide you through the path of blood sugar balance.

As you read the pages, you'll learn not only the science of blood sugar, but also how to weave lasting, healthy habits into the fabric of your everyday life. It is a guide that knows the complexities of individual experiences and pushes you to take a personalized approach to well-being—one that is in tune with your unique beat and goals.

As we start on this journey together, let "The Glucose Solution" serve as your guide, revealing the road to revolutionary blood sugar balance. Allow the tales in these pages to inspire you, the facts to strengthen you, and the practical advice to drive you toward a life of lasting energy and well-being. The adventure calls, and the answers are close at hand.

Chapter 1

Understanding Blood Sugar Basics

It's critical to understand the fundamentals that affect your health as you go on your journey to comprehend the complex dance of blood sugar inside your body. In this first part, we study the fundamentals of the dynamic world of blood sugar, which is what keeps us driven, strong, and focused.

The Pulsating Pulse of Blood Sugar

Think of your body as a well tuned symphony, with each instrument playing a specific part in keeping balance. Blood sugar is the main subject of this song, and its amounts are carefully adjusted to keep a delicate balance. Being able to notice this rhythm is important to living a happy and healthy life.

Glucose's Ascent and Decline: A Balancing Act

Even though our bodies are complex works of art, sometimes the balance slips. The rise and fall of glucose, the main figure in the blood sugar story, is studied in the opening parts of this chapter. Every step of the trip is important, from the moment you taste the first bite to the constant flow of energy.

Blood Sugar Imbalance's Effects Go Beyond Sweet Cravings

Have you ever thought why you have rapid energy slumps or strong wants for sweets? Blood sugar changes may be the hidden reason. We show how losing this fragile balance may have long-term health effects in addition to mood changes.

The Road Ahead: Getting Around the Book

It's important to set the stage for the next parts before diving further into the details of blood sugar control. We provide a plan that leads you through doable steps, expert advice, and life-changing events to help you take care of your blood sugar and change your life.

Come along on this interesting trip with us as we discover the mysteries behind blood sugar, pave the way for a transformative shift in your general health and fitness.

ideas linked to insulin, blood sugar, and how the body reacts to them.

It is crucial to comprehend the ideas of insulin and blood sugar (glucose) in order to understand the complex processes that keep the energy balance in our bodies. Let's review the fundamentals:

1. Glucose, or blood sugar:

Describe blood sugar.
Glucose, often known as blood sugar, is the main source of energy for the cells in our bodies. It comes from the food we eat, mostly from carbs. Your digestive system turns starches into glucose when you eat, which then enters your bloodstream.

Normal Blood Sugar Levels: It's important for general health to keep a normal blood sugar level. A person's regular blood sugar levels while fasting usually run from 70 to 100 mg/dL. Blood sugar levels may spike just after eating, but they should return to normal in a few hours.

Energy Source: Glucose provides energy for a range of body processes, from heavy physical exercise to basic cellular functions.

2. Insulinism:

Function of Insulin: The pancreas, an organ found under the stomach, makes the hormone insulin. Its main role is to increase glucose uptake into cells, hence controlling blood sugar levels. Following a meal, as blood sugar levels rise, the pancreas produces insulin, which tells cells to use glucose as fuel.

Insulin and Storage: Insulin is important for saving extra glucose in addition to meeting instant energy needs. It quickens the process by which extra glucose is turned into glycogen, which is kept in the muscles and liver. In times of famine or high energy demand, this saved glycogen serves as a backup that may be turned into glucose as needed.

Insulin Resistance: Insulin resistance is the word for the state that happens when cells lose their ability to respond to the effects of insulin. This leads to decreased glucose uptake by cells, which raises blood sugar levels. An important cause in the growth of type 2 diabetes is insulin resistance.

Third, Blood Sugar Control:

Homeostasis: In order to work at its peak, the body tries to keep blood sugar levels within a small range. Known as glucose homeostasis, this process needs perfect balance between insulin and other hormones that control the release of glucose from the liver and the uptake of glucose by cells.

Feedback Loop: When blood sugar levels rise after a meal, insulin is released to increase the intake of glucose. On the other hand, when there is a strong energy demand or when fasting happens, the pancreas makes less insulin, which allows the liver to release stored glucose into the bloodstream.

Making smart choices in life takes an understanding of how insulin and blood sugar combine. A healthy diet, regular exercise, and stress reduction all contribute to keeping good blood sugar levels, improving general comfort, and avoiding illnesses linked with glucose sensitivity.

How mistakes may result in health issues

Whether usually higher or uncertain, blood sugar abnormalities may have harmful effects on overall health. To keep blood sugar within a small range, the body depends on a careful balance. A change in this balance may lead to a number of health problems. Changes in blood sugar may worsen the following conditions:

1. Diabetes Type 2:

Insulin Resistance: When blood sugar levels stay high over a long length of time, cells may become less sensitive to the messages given by insulin. This is a main cause adding to the rise in type 2 diabetes.
Pancreatic exhaustion: Diabetes develops when the pancreas fails to make enough insulin to adjust for insulin resistance over time.

2. Complications linked to the heart:

Elevated blood sugar levels have been linked with a higher chance of heart disease, which includes heart attacks and strokes.
Atherosclerosis: Excessive blood sugar levels may harm blood vessels by supporting the formation of plaque, or fatty layers, which leads to atherosclerosis, a disease that blocks blood flow.

Third, Neurological Effect:

Cognitive Decline: Uncontrolled blood sugar levels have been linked with an increased chance of getting brain diseases like Alzheimer's.
Peripheral Neuropathy: Nerve damage, especially in the limbs, may result from high blood sugar. Peripheral neuropathy is marked by tingling, numbness, or pain in the hands and feet.

4. Difficulties with Weight Management:
Increased fat accumulation: Blood sugar changes may cause an increase in fat storage, especially

in the belly area. Insulin resistance and weight gain might come from this.

5. Variations in Energy and Mood:

Energy swings: Changes in blood sugar levels may lead to changes in energy levels, which can cause tiredness and anxiety.
Mood Disorders: Anxiety and sadness have been linked to bad blood sugar control.

6. Kidney Injury:

Diabetic Nephropathy: Diabetic nephropathy is a disease marked by reduced kidney function that may be brought on by repeatedly high blood sugar levels.

7. Problems with the Eyes:

Uncontrolled diabetes may grow to diabetic retinopathy, a disease that can cause blindness or vision damage by damaging the blood vessels in the eyes.

8. Inflammation Has Increased:

Inflammatory Response: Systemic inflammation is linked to a number of chronic illnesses and may be brought on by long-term changes in blood sugar levels.

9. Compromised immunological function: Weakened Immune Response: Excessive blood sugar levels may affect immunological function, increasing the body's sensitivity to diseases.

10. Pregnancy-Related Risk:

Gestational Diabetes: Blood sugar problems that form during pregnancy have the potential to become gestational diabetes, which increases the mother's and the pregnant child's risk of issues.
It is crucial to keep a healthy lifestyle that includes regular exercise, a balanced diet, and stress control in order to avoid and fix blood sugar changes. For those who are at risk or are handling blood sugar-related illnesses, regular tracking and communication with medical professionals are important.

Chapter 2

The Impact of Diet on Blood Sugar

Knowing how different meals affect blood sugar levels is crucial for anybody attempting to manage or prevent blood sugar irregularities like diabetes. Here are a few different diets and how they could affect blood sugar levels:

1. Low-Carbohydrate Diet:

Low-carb diets emphasize protein and healthy fats while limiting the amount of carbohydrates consumed.
Effect on Blood Sugar: Low-carb diets have the potential to decrease and stabilize blood sugar levels because they reduce the quantity of glucose that enters the body. Those with diabetes or insulin resistance may benefit most from this.
2. The Mediterranean Dietary Guidelines:

Full foods like fruits and vegetables, whole grains, seafood, and olive oil are emphasized in the Mediterranean diet.

Blood Sugar Effect: This diet has been associated with improved blood sugar regulation because it contains fiber, complex carbohydrates, and healthy fats. The emphasis on wholesome diet may improve insulin sensitivity.

3. Plant-Based Diet (Vegetarian or Vegan): Meals based on plants often include little to no animal products and a large amount of fruits, vegetables, legumes, nuts, and seeds.
Impact on Blood Sugar: Due to their high fiber content and low fat content, plant-based diets are often associated with improved blood sugar regulation. The high fiber content helps to maintain normal blood sugar levels by slowing the absorption of glucose.

4. Diet with Low Glycemic Index:

Foods are ranked by the glycemic index (GI) based on how they affect blood sugar levels. A low-GI diet emphasizes foods that have a lower impact on blood sugar.

Impact on Blood Sugar: Because low-GI meals raise blood glucose levels more gradually and subtly after eating, they may help regulate blood sugar.

5. Dietary Strategies to Lower Blood Pressure (DASH):

The DASH diet promotes complete meals including fruits and vegetables, lean meats, and low-fat dairy to enhance heart health.
Impact on Blood Sugar: Although the DASH diet's main goal is to control blood pressure, it may also help maintain normal blood sugar levels because of its emphasis on filling, nutrient-dense meals.
The Dietary Keto
The ketogenic diet has very little protein, a lot of fat, and very little carbohydrates. Its objective is to put the body into a state of ketosis, when it is dependent on ketones for energy.
Blood Sugar Effect: Although it may not be suitable for everyone, the ketogenic diet may drop blood sugar levels. Diabetes sufferers should continue with caution and under a physician's guidance.

Diet of the Paleolithic Period:

Full foods that our ancestors could afford, such lean meats, fish, fruits, vegetables, nuts, and seeds, are the focus of the Paleo diet.
Effects on Blood Sugar: There may be variations in the effects of the Paleo diet on blood sugar. Although it omits prepackaged meals, the outcome is determined by the dietary choices made on an individual basis.

8. Modest Diet:

Although it permits the occasional use of animal products, a flexitarian diet is mostly plant-based.
Impact on Blood Sugar: If the emphasis is on whole, raw plant foods, a flexitarian diet, like a vegetarian or vegan diet, may assist to maintain normal blood sugar levels.
Individuals may react differently to diets, therefore it's advisable to consult a medical

professional or a professional chef, particularly if you have a medical condition like diabetes. Furthermore, a person's overall way of life, meal timing, and portion size all have a significant impact on blood sugar regulation.

Useful advice for creating a diet that is blood sugar-friendly

For your diet to be healthy and blood sugar-friendly, you must choose the foods you eat carefully and in moderation. The following advice will help you create a diet that promotes stable blood sugar levels.

1. Make Whole Foods a priority:

Add a Variety of Vegetables: Try to have half of your plate consisting of non-starchy vegetables such bell peppers, broccoli, cauliflower, and leafy greens.

Select entire Fruits: Opt for entire fruits rather than fruit drinks or processed fruit snacks to increase your intake of fiber and minerals.

2. Give Priority to Complex Carbohydrates:

Whole grains, such brown rice, quinoa, oats, and whole wheat, are preferable than sweetened grains. Fiber from whole carbohydrates aids in blood sugar regulation.

Watch portion sizes: Be mindful of how much you eat and how much you consume in order to prevent severe blood sugar increases.

Third, Include Lean Proteins:

Select Lean Protein Sources: Use low-fat cheese, fish, poultry, tofu, and beans as lean protein sources in your meals. Protein increases feelings of fullness and stabilizes blood sugar.

4. Add Nutritious Fats:

Select Healthy Fats: Nuts, seeds, avocados, and olive oil are good sources of healthy fats. These fats increase feelings of fullness without significantly affecting blood sugar levels.

5. Being Mindful While Snacking:

When eating snacks, it's best to combine carbohydrates with protein or good fats to decrease their effect on blood sugar. For example, apple slices paired with peanut butter or Greek yogurt paired with berries.
Watch Out for Sugary Snacks: Eat fewer sugary snacks and more complete, nutrient-dense meals in their stead.

6. Cut Back on Added Sugars:

Check the Labels: Look for added sugars on food labels and choose those with little or no added sugar.

Natural Sweeteners: Use little amounts of natural sweeteners, such honey or maple syrup, as needed.

7. Control of Portion Size:

food control: Recognize portion sizes to avoid overindulging. To help you clearly regulate quantities, use smaller plates.
Consume Regular Foods: Keep a regular eating schedule and refrain from skipping meals, since this might alter your blood sugar levels.

Ensure Hydration:

Keep Yourself Hydrated: To keep hydrated, sip plenty of water throughout the day. Drink less sugary beverages and more water, herbal teas, or flavored water instead.

9. Include Fiber: Choose Foods High in Fiber: Increase the amount of high-fiber foods in your diet, such as whole grains, beans, and vegetables. Fiber helps to maintain normal blood sugar levels by slowing the intake of sugar.

10. Think About Meal Timing: Space Out Your Meals Throughout the Day: To prevent excessive blood sugar rises, divide your food intake among smaller, more often meals rather than large, infrequent ones.

Monitor Blood Sugar Response: You should think about monitoring your blood sugar often to observe how various meals affect you if you have diabetes or are concerned about your blood sugar levels.

11. Managing Stress:

Activities that Reduce Worry: Prolonged anxiety may affect blood sugar levels. Include stress-relieving exercises in your routine, such yoga, deep breathing, or meditation.

12. Ask a medical expert for assistance:

Seek professional assistance: To create a customized eating plan, collaborate with a medical professional or a qualified dietitian if you have diabetes or other health issues.

Keep in mind that there is no one-size-fits-all approach to a balanced diet and that individuals may react differently to various foods. These are general guidelines; it's crucial to tailor your diet to your unique requirements and health objectives.

Chapter 3

Lifestyle Changes for Blood Sugar Management

Enhancing overall health and regulating blood sugar levels both need physical activity. The following are some significant ways that exercise affects the control of blood sugar:

1. Greater Sensitivity to Insulin:

Regular exercise increases the sensitivity to insulin. Exercise reduces the overall need for insulin and aids in blood sugar regulation by making your muscles more efficient at using insulin to transfer glucose into cells.

2. Uptake of Glucose by Muscle:

During activity, muscles actively absorb glucose from the blood to use as fuel. By bringing down elevated blood sugar levels, this improves blood sugar regulation.

3. Enhanced Storage of Glycogen:

Exercise promotes the liver and muscles in particular to store more glucose as glycogen. When there is a greater need for energy, this glycogen may be released as required to assist maintain blood sugar stability.

4. Weight Management

Frequent exercise helps manage weight and may prevent or treat obesity, which is a significant risk factor for type 2 diabetes. Maintaining a healthy weight is associated with improved regulation of blood sugar.

5. Uptake of Glucose Following Exercise:

The beneficial benefits of exercise on blood sugar may last after the activity is over. After exercise, muscles continue to absorb glucose, which causes a period of elevated insulin sensitivity referred to as the "exercise effect."

There is less insulin resistance.

Insulin resistance is a condition when the body's cells lose their sensitivity to insulin signals. Exercise helps prevent this from happening. Exercise increases insulin sensitivity, which reduces the risk of type 2 diabetes.

7. Improved Heart and Vascular Health

Improved circulatory health has been associated with regular exercise. Since heart disease is one of the main consequences of diabetes, it is crucial for anybody with diabetes or at risk of developing the condition to preserve their heart health via exercise.

8. Control of Blood Pressure:

The overall health of the circulatory system depends on blood pressure regulation, which exercise may assist with. High blood pressure and diabetes often coexist, which may exacerbate their consequences.

9. Stress Reduction:

A fantastic way to relieve stress is to exercise. Prolonged anxiety may increase blood sugar levels; on the other hand, stress reduction is beneficial for blood sugar regulation and can be achieved by yoga or cardiovascular activity.

10. Better Weight Loss Sustaining:

If a person wants to lose weight and keep it off, they must exercise. Therefore, losing weight may enhance blood sugar regulation and insulin sensitivity.

Personalized Workout Plans:

Tailoring exercise regimens to each person's preferences and skill level increases adherence. Encountering enjoyable activities increases the probability of continued participation, whether it strength training, walking, riding, or a combination of these.

Consultation with Health Care Experts:

Speak with a healthcare professional to ensure the selected exercises are safe and appropriate before beginning a new fitness program, particularly for those with pre-existing health issues.

These are some suggestions for managing stress and how it affects blood sugar levels.

Blood sugar levels may be significantly impacted by stress management, which is crucial for overall health and particularly for those with diabetes or at risk for the disease.

Blood sugar levels may rise as a result of many metabolic reactions brought on by chronic anxiety. Here are some practical suggestions for managing stress and the potential effects it may have on blood sugar levels.

1. Regular Engagement in Physical Activity:

Exercise on a regular basis has been shown to be an effective stress reliever. Exercise helps regulate blood sugar and produces endorphins, the body's natural mood enhancers.

2. Mindfulness and Relaxation Techniques:

Try gradual muscle relaxation, deep breathing techniques, or mindfulness meditation to assist manage stress. These techniques could aid in fostering serenity and lessening the body's reactivity to stresses.

3. Yoga and Tai Chi:

Think about including tai chi or yoga into your regular regimen. These techniques promote serenity and reduce stress via mindfulness and physical activity.

4. Obtain Adequate Rest:

Ensure you have adequate restful sleep. Lack of sleep or poor quality of sleep may worsen stress and lower insulin sensitivity, which can raise blood sugar levels.

5. Assistance Social:

Speak with loved ones, friends, and support networks. By fostering a sense of community and providing emotional support, sharing your thoughts and experiences may help reduce stress.

6. Time Management:

Plan ahead and assign tasks to yourself. Good time management may help reduce feelings of overburden and stop anxiety from increasing.

7. Healthy Eating:

Keep up a nutritious diet. Eating meals high in nutrients may boost mood and vitality, and limiting alcohol, coffee, and sugary snacks can help maintain stable blood sugar levels.

8. Interests and free time pursuits:

Take part in activities that you like and that make you feel good. Activities for relaxation and hobbies might be useful stress relievers.

9. Set Doable Objectives:

Establish realistic objectives and break them down into manageable tasks. This technique could assist in preventing overload and lowering anxiety.

10. Develop Your Ability to Say No:

Know your own boundaries and be ready to refuse requests when necessary. Establishing boundaries is crucial to self-care since taking on too much may be stressful.

11. Look for Expert Assistance:

See a mental health professional if your concern starts to become overwhelming or persistent. Counselors and therapists may provide helpful strategies and techniques for managing stress.

12. Assess Your Blood Sugar:

Monitor the effects of concern on your blood sugar levels. Maintaining a regular monitoring schedule might assist you in identifying patterns and modifying your stress-reduction strategies accordingly.

13. Create a Calm Environment:

Establish a calm area at work or home. Make sure your surroundings are soothing, such as muted hues, pleasant scents, or dim lighting.

14. Silent Times:

Plan little moments of relaxation and rejuvenation throughout the day. Stress levels may benefit from even brief periods of relaxation.

15. Show Appreciation:

Embrace the positive aspects of your life to cultivate an attitude of gratitude. Maintaining an appreciation journal could assist you in shifting your focus and cultivating a happier outlook.

Remember that stress management is a personal journey, and that what suits one person may not suit another. Finding the strategies that are most effective for you may require some trial and error. By incorporating stress management techniques into your daily routine, you may see improvements in both your mental and blood sugar health.

Chapter 4

Meal Planning for Blood Sugar Balance

Making meals that are well-balanced is a key tactic for maintaining stable blood sugar levels. Carbs, proteins, and fats are all present in a well-balanced meal, along with fiber and important nutrients. The following rules should be adhered to when organizing meals to support stable blood sugar levels:

1. Give Proteins That Are Lean:

Every meal should contain sources of lean protein. Lean meats, fish, legumes, tofu, poultry, and low-fat dairy are a few examples.
Protein increases feelings of fullness and helps control blood sugar levels.

2. Select Intricate Carbohydrates:

Select complex carbohydrates over simple ones. Whole grains lower the risk of blood sugar spikes because they release glucose more gradually. Examples of whole grains include brown rice, quinoa, whole wheat, and oats.
Increase your intake of fiber and nutrients by including a range of vibrant vegetables.

3. Control of Portion Size:

Be mindful of portion sizes to prevent overrindulging. Reduce the size of your plates to help clearly control portions.
Think about the plate method: non-starchy vegetables should make up half of your plate, lean protein should make up one-quarter, and complex carbohydrates should make up one-quarter.

4. Add Nutritious Fats:

Nuts, seeds, avocados, and olive oil are all excellent providers of good fats. Good fats don't

affect blood sugar levels and instead encourage fullness.
Limit your intake of fat by setting a portion size limit.

5. Eat Meals High in Fiber:

Select meals high in fiber, such as whole grains, nuts, legumes, and fruits and vegetables.
Fiber helps to maintain stable blood sugar levels by slowing the absorption of glucose.

6. Mix Proteins and Fats with Carbohydrates:

Add some protein or healthy fats to your carbs to lessen their effect on blood sugar. Eat nut butter on whole grain bread or yogurt with berries, for instance.

7. Pay attention to added sugars:

Cut back on the added sugars you consume. Choose foods with minimal or no added sugars by reading food labels to determine the sources of added sugar.

Use natural sweeteners sparingly, like honey or maple syrup, if needed.

8. Consider When to Eat:

Space meals out throughout the day to prevent prolonged fasts. This aids in maintaining steady blood sugar levels.
If required, maintain energy levels between meals by including healthful snacks.

Ensure Hydration:

Drink plenty of water throughout the day. Drinking enough water is good for your body in general and can help keep your blood sugar levels steady.
Drink less sugary beverages and more water, herbal teas, or infused water instead.

10. Consume fewer processed foods:

Cut back on the amount of highly processed foods you eat, as they often include added sugars and refined carbohydrates.

Make nutrient-dense, whole foods the base of your meals.

11. Assess Response for Blood Sugar:

Keep a regular eye on your blood sugar levels to see how various meals and foods impact you. This can help you spot trends and make well-informed decisions.

12. Keep Things Uniform:

Establish a regular eating schedule with set times for meals and snacks. This consistency may help control blood sugar levels.

13. Customize to Your Unique Requirements:

Consider personal factors like age, activity level, and health conditions when organizing meals. Tailoring your strategy guarantees that the foods you choose are appropriate for your unique needs.

14. Consult a Registered Dietitian for guidance:

If you have any dietary concerns, such as diabetes, speak with a registered dietitian. They can help you create a meal plan that is tailored to your requirements and provide you with individualized advice.

15. Offer a Variety of Foods:

To make sure you receive a variety of nutrients, strive for a well-rounded and varied diet. Both blood sugar stability and general health may benefit from this.

When you follow these guidelines when meal planning, you can produce well-balanced meals that support healthy blood sugar regulation and general well-being. Since each person's response to food is unique, it can be helpful to pay attention to your body's signals and keep an eye on your blood sugar levels.

Examples of recipes and meal plans

Here are two daily meal plans that include the matching recipes.

First breakfast meal plan: breakfast bowl with quinoa and berries

One cup cooked quinoa
Half a cup of berries, including raspberries, blueberries, and strawberries
One tablespoon of nuts (walnuts or almonds) sliced
A single tsp of Greek yogurt
One tablespoon of honey
an itty bite of cinnamon
Snacking on apple slices with peanut butter

One medium apple, sliced Two tsp organic peanut butter

Lunch would be a salad and grilled chicken.

4 ounces of grilled chicken breast slices
Greens: lettuce, spinach, and arugula

Half a cup of cherry tomatoes, halved 1/4 cup of feta cheese slices, 1/4 cucumber, and a drizzle of balsamic vinegar
Berries and Greek Yogurt Snack

One cup plain Greek yogurt, two cups mixed berries, and one teaspoon chia seeds

Dinner is baked salmon, quinoa, and steamed broccoli.

baked salmon filet, six ounces
One cup of cooked quinoa
Steamed broccoli, one cup flavored with herbs and lemon

Plan 2 for Breakfast: Vegetable Omelette

Two whipped eggs
one-fourth cup diced bell peppers and one-quarter cup diced tomatoes
1/4 cup chopped spinach and 1 tsp feta cheese
Whole grain toast is optional.
Hummus on Carrot Sticks: A Snack

2 tablespoons hummus and 1 cup carrot sticks

Lunch would be soup with vegetables and lentils.

1 cup low-sodium lentil soup, either homemade or purchased from the store
mixed vegetable salad dressed with olive oil
Whole grain roll optional
As a snack, almonds and dried cranberries

one-fourth cup almonds
TWO TABLEspoONS Dried Cranberries

Dinner is Stir-fried Tofu with Brown Rice and Veggies

One cup of firm tofu cubes
One cup of mixed vegetables (bell peppers, broccoli, and snap peas) stir-fried
One cup cooked brown rice
Ginger and soy sauce as seasonings

These are just suggestions; it's important to customize them to your own dietary requirements, preferences, and any existing medical conditions. In addition, serving sizes ought to be modified in accordance with personal requirements. A registered dietitian can provide you with individualized advice if you have any specific dietary concerns.

Chapter 5

Blood Sugar and Weight Management

Blood sugar levels and weight have a complicated, reciprocal connection. Since both elements influence one another, it's essential to have a good balance for general wellbeing. The following section discusses many facets of the connection between blood sugar levels and weight:

1. Fat Storage and Insulin Resistance:

The Pancreas secretes the hormone insulin, which plays a crucial role in controlling blood sugar levels. It enhances the absorption of glucose into cells and encourages the storage of excess glucose as fat.

Insulin resistance and weight gain: Insulin resistance is a condition in which cells lose their sensitivity to insulin signals as a result of persistently elevated blood sugar levels. This might lead to elevated insulin levels, which would promote the accumulation of fat, especially around the belly.

2. Human Anatomy:

Resistance exercise is one way to maintain or gain lean body mass, which may help with blood sugar regulation and insulin sensitivity.

Overweight is associated with an increased risk of high blood sugar and insulin resistance, especially visceral fat surrounding organs.

3. Controlling blood sugar and losing weight:
Impact of Weight Loss: Reducing extra weight may enhance insulin sensitivity and improve

blood sugar regulation, particularly if the person is overweight or obese.

Diet and Exercise: It is generally advised to combine a well-balanced diet with regular physical exercise for long-term weight reduction and improved blood sugar management.

4. Obesity with Type 2 Diabetes:

Strong Correlation: A major risk factor for the development of type 2 diabetes is obesity. Impairment in glucose metabolism and insulin resistance are associated with obesity, especially abdominal fat.

Diabetes Weight Management: One of the most important aspects of controlling type 2 diabetes is keeping a healthy weight and losing weight. Blood sugar regulation may be significantly impacted by even little weight reduction.

5. The Impact of Diet:

Carbohydrate kind and Quality: Blood sugar levels may be influenced by the kind and quality of carbohydrates consumed in the diet. Diets heavy in added sugars and processed carbs may rise and fall blood sugar quickly, which may lead to weight gain.

Protein and Fiber: Consuming enough amounts of these nutrients in the diet may help control blood sugar levels, encourage satiety, and aid in weight management.

Syndrome Metabolic (MS):
Metabolic syndrome, a collection of disorders that includes elevated blood pressure, elevated blood sugar, and abnormal lipid levels, is often linked to obesity. The two main treatments for metabolic syndrome are diet and lifestyle modifications.

7. Stress and Cortisol:
Stress Response: Prolonged stress may cause insulin resistance and weight gain by increasing cortisol levels.

Stress Management: Practicing stress-reduction strategies like mindfulness, consistent exercise, and getting enough sleep will help lower blood sugar and promote weight loss.

Individual Variations
The way the body reacts to changes in weight and blood sugar regulation may be influenced by individual genetic characteristics.

Individual Responses to Dietary and Lifestyle treatments: It is important to stress the relevance of tailored approaches to blood sugar control and weight management by acknowledging that people may respond differently to dietary and lifestyle treatments.

9. Drugs and Increased Weight:
Some drugs: Weight gain may result from using some drugs to treat diabetes or other medical disorders. It's essential to talk to your doctor about any possible weight implications.

Loop of Positive Feedback 10:
Positive Weight Changes: By enhancing insulin sensitivity and blood sugar regulation, positive weight changes, such as weight loss achieved via healthy lifestyle modifications, may provide a positive feedback loop.

For the purpose of managing diabetes and controlling weight, it is essential to comprehend the connection between blood sugar levels and weight. A good balance of blood sugar levels and weight may be attained and maintained by a variety of strategies, including stress management, regular exercise, a balanced diet, and receiving enough sleep. You should get individualized guidance from a healthcare provider if you have particular concerns about your weight or blood sugar levels.

Techniques for controlling blood sugar that can help you reach and stay at a healthy weight.

Blood sugar control and reaching and maintaining a healthy weight are closely related, especially for those who already have diabetes or are at risk of getting it. These are a few tactics that combine blood sugar regulation with weight reduction.

Blood sugar control and reaching and maintaining a healthy weight are closely related, especially for those who already have diabetes or are at risk of getting it. The following are some methods that combine blood sugar regulation with weight loss:

A diet that is well-balanced:
Eating a diet rich in whole foods, such as fruits, vegetables, whole grains, lean meats, and healthy fats, is recommended.

Restrict Portion Sizes: Restricting portion sizes might help you cut down on calories. Utilize resources like the plate approach to guarantee a nutritional distribution that is balanced.

2. Control of Carbohydrates:

Make Complex carbs a Priority: Low-GI complex carbs include legumes, whole grains, and non-starchy vegetables.

Spread Your Carbohydrate Intake Throughout the Day: Distribute your carbohydrate intake equally throughout the day to prevent significant blood sugar increases.

3. Intake of Protein:

Lean Proteins: Consume foods high in lean protein, such as fish, chicken, tofu, lentils, and reduced-fat dairy. Protein promotes fullness and may prevent overindulging.

4. Healthy Fats:

Select Good Fats: Nuts, seeds, avocados, and olive oil are excellent sources of healthy fats. Aim to limit total calorie consumption by paying attention to portion sizes.

5. High-Fibre Foods:

Add foods high in fiber, such as legumes, whole grains, fruits, and vegetables. In addition to helping to regulate blood sugar, fiber also increases feelings of fullness.

6. Regular Engagement in Physical Activity:

Combine Strength and Aerobic Training: Mix activities that target both strength and cardio (e.g., walking, running, swimming). Exercise promotes weight reduction and increases insulin sensitivity.

Being consistent is crucial. Aim for twice-weekly strength training in addition to at least 150 minutes of moderate-intensity aerobic exercise per week.

7. Managing Weight:

Weigh-Ins: Weigh yourself often to monitor your progress. But instead of concentrating only on the scale's number, think about general health gains.

8. Meal Planning:

Meal Schedule: Make sure your mealtimes are consistent and on a regular basis. Avoid missing meals to prevent blood sugar swings.

9. Stress Management:

Incorporate Activities That Relieve Stress: Engaging in stress-relieving activities like deep breathing, yoga, meditation, or hobbies is recommended. Prolonged stress might cause weight gain and increase blood sugar levels.

10. Obtain Adequate Sleep:

Make Getting Enough Good Sleep a Priority: Ensure that each night you receive enough good sleep. Hormones that regulate appetite and satiety may be upset by sleep loss, which may result in weight gain.

11. Beverages

Drink Water Throughout the Day: you keep hydrated, be sure you regularly consume water. Occasionally, the body confuses thirst for hunger, leading to an overindulgence in calories.

12. Customized Method:

Seek Professional Advice: If you suffer from diabetes or any other health issue, speak with a certified dietitian or endocrinologist for individualized guidance.

13. Administration of Medication:

Recognize Medication implications: Be mindful of any possible weight implications if you take diabetic medication. Consult your physician about any worries or modifications.

14. Modifications in Behavior:

Determine Triggers: Acknowledge the psychological or environmental cues that cause unhealthful eating patterns, and endeavor to create more constructive coping strategies.

15. Gradient Changes:

Sustainable Lifestyle adjustments: Aim for long-term, progressive adjustments rather than quick fixes. This promotes sustained dedication to a healthy way of living.

16. Helping Hands:

Establish a Support System: Encircle yourself with a family, friends, or medical team that will be there for you when you need them. Reaching and maintaining a healthy weight may be facilitated by accountability and encouragement.

Since everyone responds differently to techniques, customize these suggestions to your own requirements and situation. Patience and consistency are key when it comes to controlling blood sugar levels and losing weight. Always ask medical specialists for their specific counsel and advise.

Chapter 6

Special Considerations: Blood Sugar and Specific Groups

Physiological changes, lifestyle choices, and personal health concerns all affect how blood sugar is regulated in different populations. This is a summary of how pregnant women, the elderly, and teenagers manage their blood sugar:

1. Children:

The growth and development of children need the consumption of certain nutrients. Maintaining blood sugar regulation is essential to provide them with the energy they need, especially during times of fast growth.

Snacking and Meal Timing: Children may benefit from regular meal and refreshment times to maintain stable blood sugar levels. Long-term energy requires a variety of macronutrients found in balanced meals.

Exercise: It's critical to motivate teenagers to participate in regular physical activity. It supports blood sugar management in addition to overall wellness.

Parental Guidance: In especially for children with conditions like type 1 diabetes, parents are crucial in ensuring that their children follow a balanced diet, set up good eating habits, and control their blood sugar levels.

2. Older people:

Insulin Sensitivity: It has been shown that insulin sensitivity declines with age. Seniors who consume high amounts of carbohydrates should reduce their intake to prevent blood sugar spikes.

Nutrient Absorption: It's possible for some older people to have trouble absorbing nutrients. Maintain a diet high in nutrients, and if necessary, think about taking supplements.

prescription adjustments: Older people on diabetes drugs may need prescription adjustments due to differences in metabolism and renal function. Regular monitoring and consultation with medical professionals are essential.

Well-Balanced Meals: Increasingly, maintaining blood sugar levels and overall health depends on eating a diet rich in whole foods.

3. Mothers-to-be:

Pregnancy is the primary cause of gestational diabetes, a kind of the disease. Maintaining blood sugar management is essential to preventing problems for the mother and the child.

Nutrient Needs: Pregnancy increases the body's need for certain nutrients, and blood sugar regulation is essential to avoiding complications related to gestational diabetes and excessive weight gain.

It may be necessary for expectant mothers with gestational diabetes to periodically check their blood sugar levels. In certain cases, medication or insulin therapy may be given under a doctor's supervision.

Postpartum Considerations: Since gestational diabetes increases the risk of acquiring type 2 diabetes later in life, blood sugar management is crucial after delivery.

4. Socioeconomic and cultural factors

Dietary patterns: Access to healthcare, lifestyle decisions, and eating habits may be influenced by cultural and socioeconomic factors. Providing adequate blood sugar management solutions requires an understanding of and tolerance for cultural differences.

Community Support: Education and community support are crucial to addressing blood sugar management in a variety of groups. Interventions with a specific cultural context in mind could work better.

5. Tailored Care:

Any demographic may be affected by underlying health conditions that affect the control of blood sugar. Examples of this include hormone abnormalities, kidney disease, and cardiovascular diseases. Customizing care to each patient's unique health profile is essential.

Changes in lifestyle factors that impact blood sugar include physical activity, stress levels, and sleep habits. It is essential to address each of these issues separately in order to manage effectively.

6. Technology and Tools:

Monitoring monitors: People of all ages may benefit greatly from technological advancements like continuous glucose monitoring monitors. Yet, there may be differences in such technology uptake and accessibility.

7. Healthcare Access:

Access to Healthcare: Inequalities in this area may make it more difficult for people from different demographic groups to get timely and effective treatment. To properly control blood sugar, these discrepancies must be resolved.

Counsel suited for certain demographics

Let's provide certain populations—like teenagers, the elderly, and pregnant mothers—individualized advice.

Healthy Snacks and Meals for Kids:

Make certain that kids' meals include a range of healthy fats, proteins, and carbs.
Promote regular, well-planned snacking to prevent blood sugar swings.

Nutrient-Dense Foods: Give priority to nutrient-dense foods in order to promote growth and development.
Incorporate supplies of vitamins, iron, and calcium into their diet.

saccharine munchies: Reduce the amount of drinks and saccharine munchies you consume.
Select nutritious alternatives like yogurt, nuts, or fruits.

Regularly promote leisure and physical activity.

Limit screen usage and promote outdoor recreation.

Parental Involvement: Parents need to keep a close eye on and provide direction for their kids' eating habits.
Instill in them the importance of eating a balanced diet.

Nutritional Guidelines for Seniors:

Stress the importance of eating a balanced diet full of veggies, lean meats, and nutritious cereals.
You should think about eating smaller, more often meals to help reduce blood sugar levels.

Drink plenty of water since dehydration might affect blood sugar levels.
Stay away from sugary drinks and stick to water or herbal infusions.

Frequent Blood Sugar Monitoring: Especially if you have diabetes, be sure to regularly check your blood sugar levels.

In reaction to variations in blood sugar, modify your medication and food.

Nutrient Absorption: To improve bone health, eat a diet high in calcium and vitamin D.
Speak with a medical professional about potential vitamin supplements.

Physical Activity: Adapt activities to individual capabilities and regularly engage in moderate-intensity exercise.
Exercise may help with weight management and raise insulin sensitivity.

Handling Gestational Diabetes in Expectant Mothers:

Regular monitoring of blood sugar levels is recommended, especially if you have gestational diabetes.
Observe the dietary recommendations suggested by your medical professional.

It is advised to follow a balanced diet that meets the infant's and mother's nutritional needs.
Add supplies of calcium, iron, and folic acid.

Meal Timing: To assist control your blood sugar levels, space out your meals throughout the day. If need, think about eating in smaller, more frequent quantities.

Prenatal Care: Pay attention to your doctor's advise and schedule frequent prenatal checkups. Deal with any issues or modifications to blood sugar regulation as soon as it is practical.

Recommendations Following Childbirth: After giving birth, keep an eye on your blood sugar levels, especially if you were diagnosed with gestational diabetes.

Make sustained, incremental lifestyle adjustments your top priority for long-term health.

Customized Methods: Overarching Ideas for Every Group:

Dietary and lifestyle recommendations should be customized for each person based on their preferences and health issues.
When formulating dietary recommendations, take personal and cultural factors into account.

Regular testing of blood sugar levels should be done as prescribed by medical professionals.
Keep a record of your food intake, exercise routine, and any notable adjustments.

Advice from Healthcare Professionals: Speak with doctors and dietitians to get personalized guidance.
Adjust the plan in response to regular health assessments and professional advice.

Achieve total blood sugar regulation by addressing lifestyle factors including stress, sleep, and exercise.

Conclusion

We find ourselves at a crossroads in the last chapters of "The Glucose Solution: A Guide to Transformative Blood Sugar Balance," when knowledge combines with empowerment and information meets action. This trip through the intricate network of blood sugar dynamics has been an educational experience that now points us in the direction of a future shaped by deliberate living and well-informed decision-making.

Let us take away from these pages the profound knowledge that our bodies are intricate symphonies, with our daily choices acting as the notes representing our health. Let us bid these pages farewell. Blood sugar's long-mysterious dance is now one we can direct with focus and intention.

"The Glucose Solution" is not a finish line, but rather the beginning of an enduring relationship with your health. It enables you to embrace the ups and downs of your path toward health, understanding that it's not about limitation but about development, and that perfection is not the goal.

Remember this as you go forward, equipped with the concepts presented in these pages: revolutionary change is a mosaic made up of the little, deliberate pieces that make up our routines and decisions. Honor the victories, take lessons from the setbacks, and welcome the never-ending journey toward a harmonious and fulfilling life.

I hope the stories, insights, and useful advice in this book continue to resonate in your daily life and serve as a guide for you as you traverse the complexities of today's world. Allow the path to blood sugar homeostasis to serve as a trigger for general health, creating a domino effect that permeates every aspect of your existence.

You are the protagonist, the writer, and the artist in the amazing tapestry that is your health. "The Glucose Solution" is only a roadmap, a collaborator in your pursuit of optimal well-being. May you carry the torch of knowledge, the flame of self-awareness, and the light of empowerment into the chapters of your life that remain to be written as you close this book. May the transforming energy that is within you be seen by your well-being, your path being illuminated, and your choices being deliberate. The best parts are still to come, as the voyage keeps going.